Gaming Hunger

Better Health with Sugar Detox and Intermittent Fasting

Samuel Tyuluman, M.D.

ISBN-13:9781731306470

DEDICATION

To Mrs. Moss
The most wonderful 4th grade teacher ever!!

CONTENTS

ACKNOWLEDGMENTS

Productions Editor: Chelsea Chapman Illustrator: Adam
Walker
Cover: "New Horizon" Image - National Space Society
Founder: Wernher von Braun

SECTION 1
HOUSTON!
WE HAVE A BIG PROBLEM

Five years ago, my cardiologist told me to "lose a few pounds". Like 45 pounds!!   But he had no idea how I should do it. He wanted me to start statins to lower my cholesterol. My A1c was nearly 6 (pre-diabetic). I was eating low fat and exercising every day. I didn't feel like I was over eating. The statins made my muscles ache. Then I heard about intermittent fasting on a public radio show. The talk was about the 5-2 fast, so I got the book, read it and got started. The "5-2" diet allows up to 500 calories a day, but not more than that on a fasting day. You "fast" two days a week, that's where the name comes from, fast 2 days eat as usual 5 days. It was mostly a cook book with recipes that had less than 500 calories. It was a diet - counting calories, watching my weight... yada, yada, yada...

It didn't work.

Besides, I didn't want to "watch my weight" - I wanted to control it! AND lower my risk for heart disease and diabetes. Months went by without any changes. I wondered why it wasn't working. Then I found tons of research on Ghrelin and Leptin, literally tons of it! – The program for Sugar Detox and Intermittent Fasting was born – It works, it is a Design for Wellness; not a diet, but a lifestyle change...

In over 30 years of patient consultations - by far the dominant question was how to lose weight. I've seen some very expensive, dangerous and bizarre programs over the years. None of them worked permanently. Intermittent fasting, done correctly, has shown to be the one method of getting control over your weight, permanently. As you will see, it also has some other very, very positive health benefits. But first a little background about our nutrition in the United States.

The food in this country makes us hungry and prone to overeating. In effect, the food we eat drives us to eat more, leading to obesity, insulin resistance and diabetes. In United States alone 300,000 people die each year from obesity-related diseases. In the United States, type two diabetes mellitus (T2DM) is epidemic. The Center for Disease Control (CDC) estimates that over 8% of the population suffer from T2DM. It is rapidly becoming a disease in younger and younger people [6]. Diabetes causes serious diseases like kidney failure, lower-limb amputations, and blindness. Type two diabetes is associated with Alzheimer's disease ("Type 3 Diabetes"). We have gone from a stable 3.5 diabetics per 100 patients in 1996 to 9/100 in 2015. And this number is still rising – rapidly. The first step in turning this epidemic around is education. One person at a time if need be.

Since the mid 1970's when high fructose corn syrup (HFCS) was declared "Safe" by the FDA and used in the U.S. as a sweetener the incidence of insulin resistance (T2DM) and obesity has increased. Not only is HFCS considered safe by the FDA, the production of HFCS is subsidized by the U.S. government [19]. HFCS plays a major role in this American epidemic of obesity. Consequently, by the mid 1980's we became an obese population searching for the "right diet"; the Adkins Diet, the Keto Diet, the Paleo Diet. The stomach is under attack with gastric bands, gastric balloons gastric sleeves and gastric bypasses are marketed everywhere. The stomach is not the source of the problem. Far from it.

Obesity, T2DM and Alzheimer's Disease all share a common cause: insulin resistance, a consequence of excessive sugar intake. Diets and bariatric surgeries won't fix insulin resistance - only a lifestyle change can to that. Designs For Wellness helps you understand the causes for insulin resistance and provides you with treatments and lifestyle changes that will reduce insulin resistance, give you control over your weight and improve your overall health. Understanding the driving forces behind this obesity epidemic will make it easier for you to create your Design For Wellness, one that fits you.

SECTION 2
THE HUNGER GAME
HUNGER FOR PROFIT

Other things contribute to obesity like over eating and a sedentary lifestyle, but, clearly, high fructose corn syrup (HFCS) is a major contributing factor in this obesity epidemic. I will lay out the link between the use of fructose, increased sugar consumption and obesity [7-9]. In the U.S., the food industry argues that HFCS is easier to handle than granulated sugar which is 50% glucose - 50% fructose. In 1976 the U.S. Food and Drug Administration classified HFCS as G.R.A.S., "Generally Recognized as Safe" and high fructose corn syrup (HFCS) replaced granulated sugar as a sweetener [15]. HFCS is THE sweetener in soft drinks manufactured in the U.S. HFCS isn't used much in any other countries. Soft drink makers, Coca-Cola and Pepsi, are the biggest producers of soft drinks in world and in the U.S., they use nothing but HFCS to sweeten their soft drinks [18]. Large Agra-corporations, such as Archer Daniels Midland, successfully lobby for government corn subsidies (corn being the source for HFCS) [19], even though fructose is known to increase appetite, body weight, insulin resistance, and T2DM. The European Union does not recognize HFCS as safe and, therefore, obesity is not nearly as prevalent there as it is in the United States. The people of the EU do enjoy sweets, but they use a different sweetener, granulated sugar. The EU consumed 18.6 million tons of granulate sugar every year between 1999- 2005 [17] but, the production of HFCS in the EU was only 303 thousand tons in 2005. They simply don't consider HFCS safe for their population and don't have much use for it. Fructose **stimulates** appetite and that, of course, **stimulates** the sales of foods that **stimulate** appetite and that **stimulates** the... Well, you get the point here.

The obesity epidemic in the U.S. is not due to our weakness, but to the addictive nature of our food; those foods and drinks containing fructose make you want to eat more. The world seems to know that HFCS promotes obesity (massive, morbid obesity) and associated chronic diseases, yet the U.S. government continues to label high fructose corn syrup as Generally Regarded As Safe (GRAS) and subsidize its production.

SECTION 3
COMMON WEIGHT LOSS MEASURES

The Ketogenic Diet - In 3-4 days of ZERO carbohydrate intake, fat is turned, not into sugar, but into ketone bodies which can be used in place of sugar. Reducing sugar intake decreases the need for excessive production of insulin, which reduces insulin resistance and yields many health benefits, including a significant reduction in heart disease. The ketogenic diet as healthy as it is, is hard to maintain and is still only a temporary measure for the treatment of obesity. It is not a lifestyle change. The ketogenic diet takes a conscious, strict, and highly disciplined, daily commitment. One carbohydrate containing meal throws you out of ketosis. Since carbohydrate (especially fructose) is in just about everything, staying in ketosis is a real tough challenge. Bariatric surgery started in the 1950s while gastric bypass was not used until 1965. Today, bariatric surgery reduces the size of the stomach, this stops Ghrelin release earlier in a meal. Ghrelin is the hormone made by the stomach that drives the appetite. Unfortunately, over 90% of these surgeries fail because, without a change in eating habits, the stomach stretches out again and Ghrelin production goes back to pre-surgery levels.

The gastric balloon is another attempt to control the release of Ghrelin. A balloon stretches out the stomach, preventing the release of Ghrelin, so there is less of an appetite. The use of balloons started in 1938. In 1985, the Garren-Edwards Bubble was approved by the FDA but withdrawn seven years later because of lethal complications. The FDA approved a new balloon in 2015 but deaths are already being reported. This desperate method of weight loss reduces the release of Ghrelin, reducing appetite. When the balloon is removed Ghrelin production goes back normal levels and appetite and obesity return just as before. Ghrelin is a hormone that does more than drive appetite, a lot more. Among other things it releases growth hormone, improves memory, and problem solving. So, instead of cutting out the production of Ghrelin, Designs For Wellness teaches patients how to use Ghrelin to improve their health. Teaching patients about their bodies takes more time, is more labor intensive and produces less revenue, but results in a safer, much more positive, permanent, and effective change for the life of our patients.

SECTION 4
GETTING YOUR BALANCE BACK

Understanding how hunger and satiety work goes a long way toward making this lifestyle change effective and permanent. Our brain has an impulse-receiving center, the hypothalamus, which gets signals from all over the body. These signals provoke behaviors from fighting to appetite to sexual behavior. The hormone Ghrelin, is the "eat or die" hormone, released from the stomach when it is empty. Leptin, is the "stop eating or die" hormone that is released from fat. They both go to the brain and fight it out in the hunger game. Ghrelin is short for "Growth Hormone RELeasing INitiator", Leptin is Greek for "thin". We had no idea that these hormones had anything to do with growth hormone release or appetite control prior to 1994 (Leptin), 1995 (Ghrelin) When your stomach is empty, Ghrelin, the "eat or die" hormone, pumps out and the brain gets the signal that you must eat, NOW. Ghrelin is released until the stomach is stretched [Figure 1].

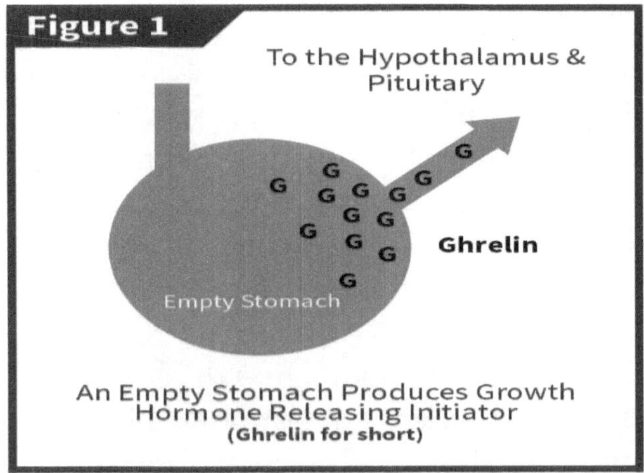

An Empty Stomach Produces Growth Hormone Releasing Initiator
(Ghrelin for short)

Ghrelin is a must during infancy. A baby cannot even crawl to get milk for months after birth. It must get the attention of its mom - or just lay there and waste away. The baby's Ghrelin is released from the stomach, goes to the brain giving an infant a very, very intense drive to feed. Ghrelin makes the baby produce a LOT OF NOISE until it's stomach is stretched. [Figure 2].

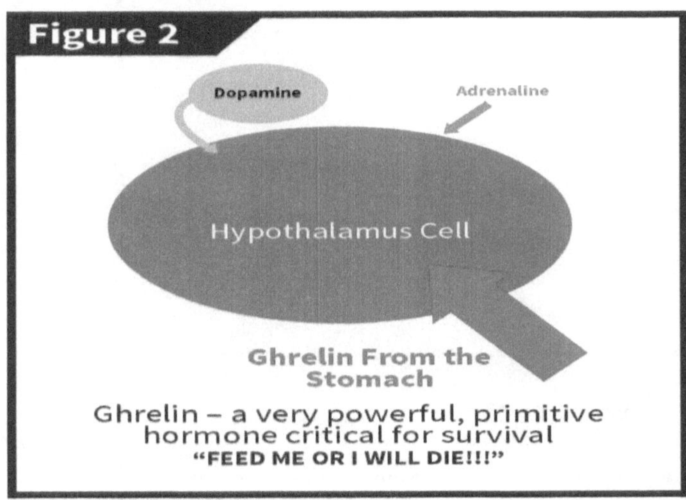

Ghrelin – a very powerful, primitive hormone critical for survival
"FEED ME OR I WILL DIE!!!"

Without Ghrelin, a baby will not survive. The hormone Ghrelin is released by the stomach throughout life. When part of the stomach is removed during bariatric surgery, Ghrelin is decreased, and the appetite is decreased. As the stomach stretches again, Ghrelin production increases and appetite increases. To begin with, Ghrelin, as we will see, and as the name implies, causes the release of human growth hormone (HGH), a LOT of human growth hormone, 20 times the normal levels of HGH. This crucial release of HGH happens only one time during a fast, no matter how long the fast lasts. [31]. Leptin, meaning "thin" in Greek, brings on satisfaction calling an end to the meal, it is the "satiety" hormone. Leptin blunts the effects of Ghrelin. Leptin is produced by white fat; the jiggly stuff we all hate [Figure 3].

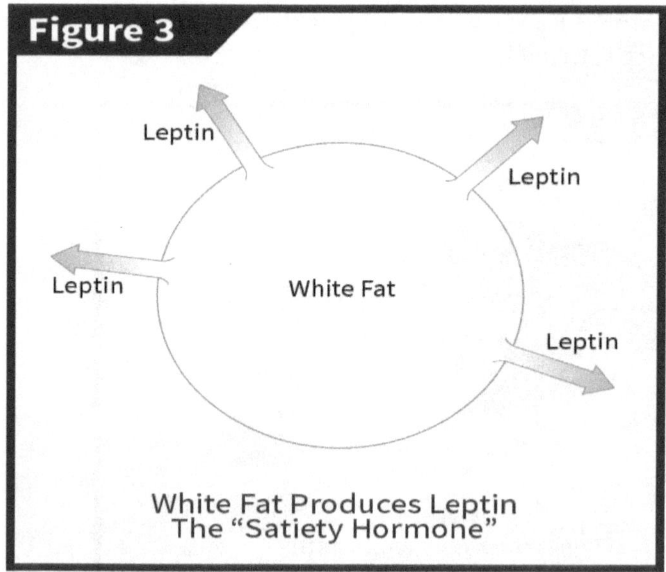

Just as an infant would waste away without Ghrelin, an obese child is at a tremendous disadvantage. To survive and reproduce, it is very important to outrun the slowest member of the tribe. This makes both Ghrelin and Leptin very important survival hormones - in the wild if this balance is disturbed, survival is threatened. The bottom line is; without Leptin or Ghrelin, and the brilliant partnership of the two, an individual would not survive long enough to reproduce in the wild. Leptin and Ghrelin create the "set point" of our body weight [Figure 4]. Leptin blocks the effects of Ghrelin in the cells of the brain, suppressing appetite, "shrinking the stomach".

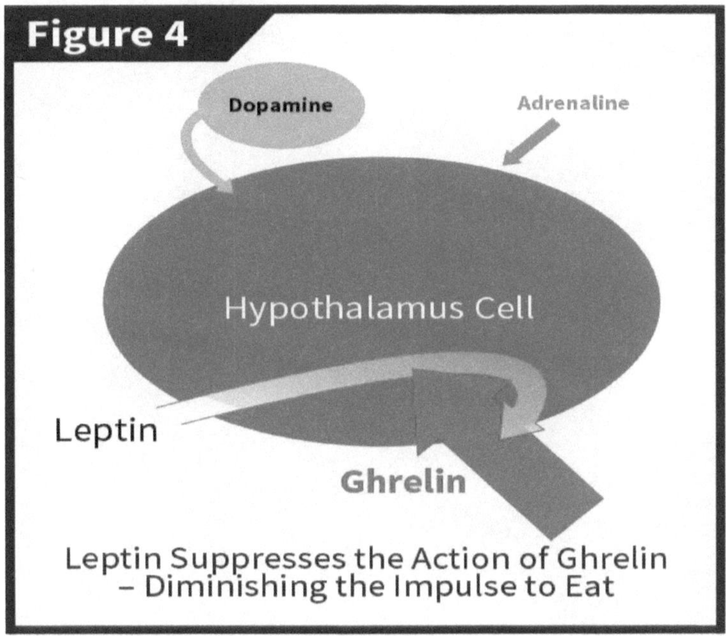

Samuel Tyuluman

12

SECTION 5
GHRELIN'S GONE WILD

The lead article in the New England Journal of Medicine (January 2015) demonstrated the effects of uncontrolled Ghrelin and the impact Leptin has on hunger and obesity. This otherwise healthy German child of Turkish descent was born without functional Leptin, a very rare condition [Figure 5].

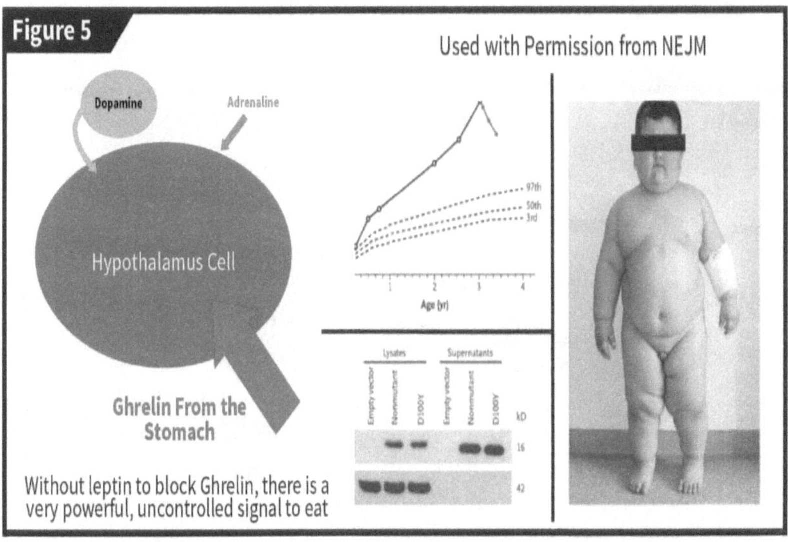

From birth this child needed to have his stomach filled almost every hour. He would eat as much as 600 calories per feeding. If denied food, he would eat anything that would stretch his stomach and stop the Ghrelin release. At three times normal weight just before his 3rd birthday, he was eating himself to death. Once the problem was diagnosed, and Leptin injections were administered, this behavior stopped. He was more easily satisfied and began to return to a normal, healthy weight. Keep in mind he was in Germany where fructose is not a staple. As normal humans, we have normal Leptin and Ghrelin. The big problem for Americans is fructose; it is a staple in our diet. Fructose (HFCS) prevents the release of Leptin from fatty tissue and it prevents Leptin from getting into the brain, which means Ghrelin goes wild just as with the Leptin Baby. You just "can't get no satisfaction", no satiety [Figure 6].

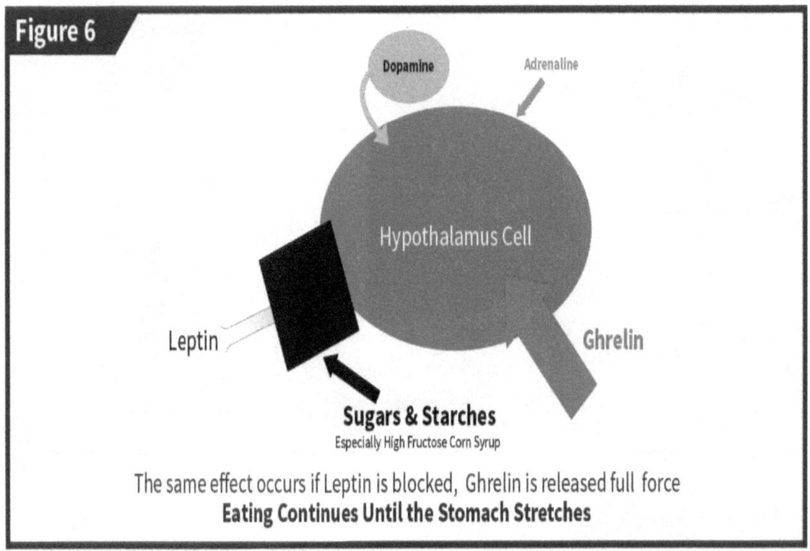

We may as well not even produce Leptin. High Fructose Corn syrup is a great Leptin blocker and rampant obesity, insulin resistance and diabetes are the result. Since the Leptin and Ghrelin interact only inside the cells of the brain, the amount of Leptin circulating in the blood doesn't matter. If fructose blocks Leptin, Ghrelin, the powerful appetite stimulating hormone, goes completely wild. Buying and taking extra Leptin won't work, since any Leptin will be blocked from getting into the brain no matter where it comes from. The morbidly obese have plenty of Leptin but its effects are blocked. As the stomach is stretched larger and larger, it produces more and more Ghrelin, making Leptin less and less effective, increasing the volume of food required to stop Ghrelin release. This is a vicious cycle that will not stop until either the Leptin block is removed or Ghrelin is allowed to do what it was intended to do. To counter this and stop the slide into obesity, Design For Wellness recommends two measures.

1. Get as much fructose (HFCS) and carbohydrates out of the diet as possible and allow Leptin to do its job. It is not necessary to remove all carbohydrates (ketogenic diet) if Leptin is still able to do its job balancing Ghrelin.

2. Consider using the insulin sensitizer, Metformin. Use it as an appetite suppressant, to reduce insulin resistance and allow Leptin to enter the brain.

SECTION 6
THE FRENCH LILAC - METFORMIN

Metformin's role in the treatment of obesity and weight management is reducing Leptin block. Metformin is an appetite suppressant, because it opens the path for Leptin to get into the brain. This leads to reduced appetite and control over the effects Ghrelin [Figure 7]. Unlike newer weight loss medications and appetite suppressants, Metformin suppresses appetite, but it will do it with fewer side effects and at a much lower cost. In addition it has other very positive effects on health and longevity; cancer risk reduction, and possibly a decreased risk for dementia. Metformin has a safety profile better than aspirin. Metformin is on the World Health Organizations Model List of Essential Medicines (19th List) [30].

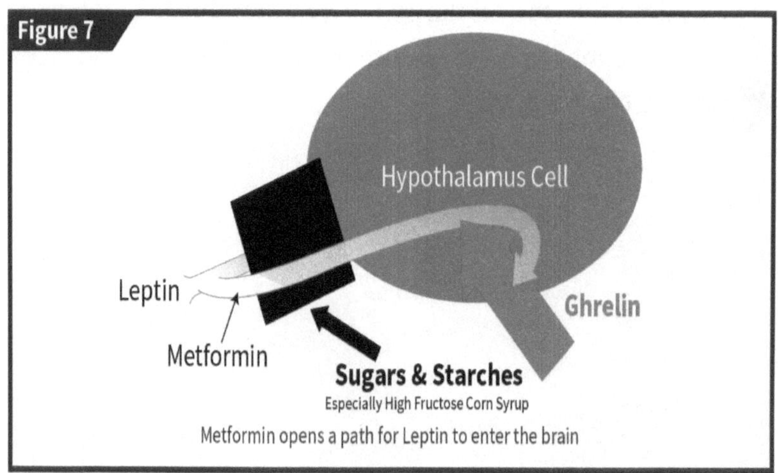

Metformin remains one of the most commonly prescribed drugs in the world with nearly 120 million prescriptions filled yearly worldwide [26]. Metformin was approved for the treatment of diabetes in Britain in 1958, Canada in 1972, and the US in 1995. In addition to treating diabetes, Dr. Tyuluman, M.D., founder of Designs For Wellness, has used Metformin off label to treat the infertility caused by the polycystic ovary syndrome (PCOs) since 1995 and obesity since 2007. Both conditions are associated with high levels of insulin resistance.

Many of the PCOS infertility patients lost weight and requested to continue to use Metformin as an appetite suppressant. We have used metformin "off label" for these patients since 1995, we have seen no significant side effects, other than stomach upset, which resolves with time and improved diet. There is also a lot of research regarding Metformin and its role in the prevention of pre-eclampsia, cancer [24,27-29] and dementia [20,26] The medication, Metformin comes from the French lilac [Figure 8] and was used for the treatment of type 2 diabetes and mental illness by ancient Egyptian physicians and doctors in medieval Europe [22,23]. The wholesale price of Metformin throughout the world was between US$0.21 and US$5.55 per month as of 2014. Metformin, however, is not for everyone. A patient must have normal kidneys and should not take Metformin before major surgery or X-rays that require contrast. Metformin must always be prescribed by a physician. Dr. Tyuluman has more than 20 years' experience prescribing Metformin for polycystic ovarian syndrome, type 2 diabetes, weight management and other conditions caused by insulin resistance. Metformin is a very useful and safe preventive medicine.

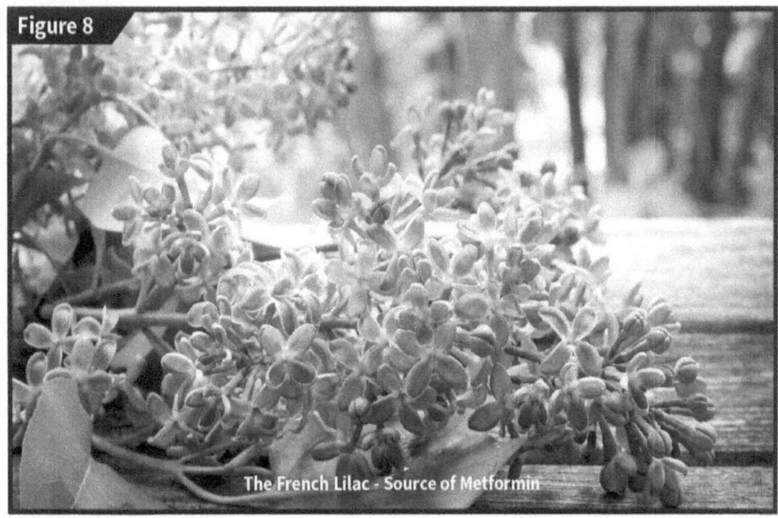

SECTION 7
WAIT!!! MY WEIGHT??

"I work out like crazy and eat low carb but I cannot get this extra weight off! Why?"

This has everything to do with the way fat is stored. Your body has two kinds of fat; brown fat - it's almost sugar and almost fat and white fat - the stuff that jiggles and won't easily go away. Adults have a 1/2 pound "compartment" of brown fat that is kept near your brain since your brain burns sugar like crazy. Everyone has ½ pound of brown fat stored at any time. Brown fat keeps blood sugar at 100mg/dl. Brown fat keeps the blood glucose very tightly regulated. It provides the fuel for your brain, muscles, your temperature regulation, heartbeat, breathing, and thinking [Figure 9].

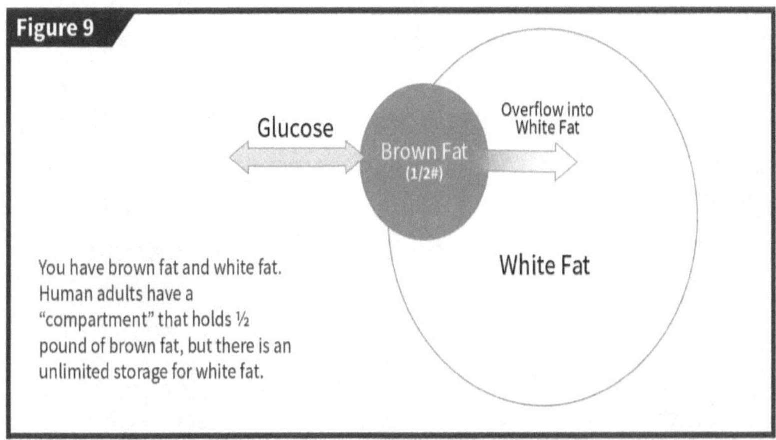

White fat is like a protected bin of stored energy. It's like your "401K of energy". You can't burn white fat, you must turn it into ketone bodies (the "keto diet") to use it for energy. Since you cannot instantly turn white fat into usable sugar, you must have enough brown fat to keep sugar levels normal and to keep your brain working, your heart pumping and your temperature regulated. Very little sugar is circulating in the blood at any given time and it is very tightly regulated; too much gives you diabetes, too little results in a coma. Since ketosis is days away, if you run out of brown fat too quickly, you are in real trouble. White fat is used for energy in only two special circumstances:

1. When the body is in ketosis

2. In response to a big pulse of human growth hormone (HGH)

A ½ pound of fat will carry you about 25 miles or last you about 24 hours without being restored by a meal. Since a human only has about ½ pound of brown fat to burn and exercise does not turn white fat into sugar, it is not surprising that the distance for the Olympic marathon has been 26.2 miles since the time of the Ancient Greeks. It tests the upper limits, and beyond, of the human athlete. A normal human is not capable of running much further than 25 miles [Figure 10] without complete exhaustion. Only very, very special people, the "Olympian", can go that extra 1.2 mile.

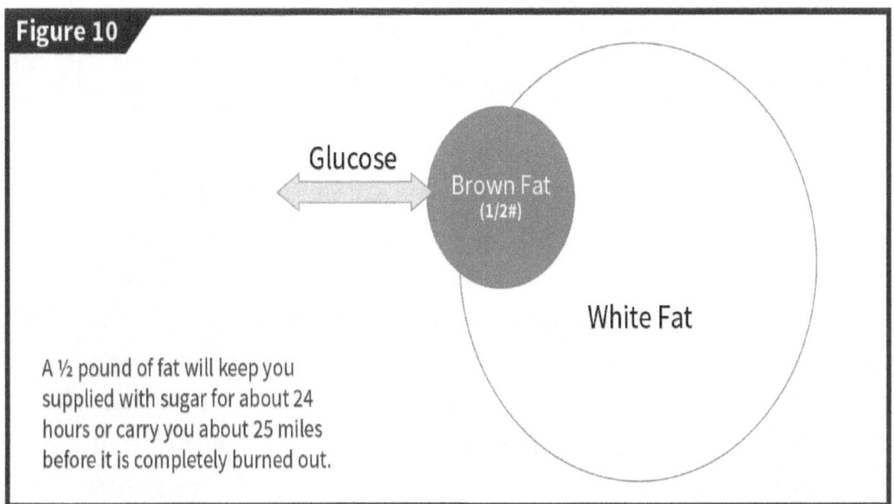

In modern times, marathoner's carb load and take in oral glucose along the way.   If they didn't, they'd either fail to complete the race, or they'd die trying…   But what about fasting? - It burns away brown fat.   Just like the runner, it is gone in 24 hours, but we don't become exhausted or lay down and die? People can go days without eating. Ketosis (starvation mode) does not happen for some 2-3 days?   How can we survive this day or two before we go into starvation mode ketosis?

SECTION 8
THE LOGIC OF
INTERMITTENT FASTING

If your brown fat will take you 25 miles or about 24 hours without food, if a human will collapse at the end of a 25-mile run when the brown fat burns out, how can humans survive without food for days?? Ketosis is days away. Not an uncommon situation at all.

Ghrelin!!! Yes, the hormone that has been cut out of stomachs and suppressing since 1965! Ghrelin helps you to survive this transition by triggering one big dump of human growth hormone. This pulse of growth hormone converts ½ pound of white fat into brown fat (glucose) which can be used right away as an energy source. This is the only time white fat is turned directly into sugar, reversing fat storage. A successful fast turns 1/2 pound of white fat into sugar (glucose) for immediate use by the body. Without this boost in brown fat it would be impossible to maintain breathing, temperature, heart beat or brain function until ketosis (starvation) begins. The hormone Ghrelin also works to reduce inflammatory reactions, improves memory and attention span, it even has antidepressant effect. Ghrelin is extensively woven into many signals and processes of the body. Artificially cutting production of Ghrelin has far reaching negative effects on health and wellbeing. For this reason,

Designs For Wellness strongly discourages bariatric surgery. Ghrelin's dominant role is, as its name implies- Growth Hormone RELeasing INitiator Ghrelin is released from the stomach when the stomach is empty, and the signal is pulsed continuously to the pituitary until the stomach is stretched. Studies conducted as far back as 1988 [31] show that there is a dump of twenty times the normal level of Human Growth Hormone (HGH) between 16-24 hours of continuous fasting. This release of HGH only happens once during a fast no matter how long the fasting goes on. Continued fasting beyond the first HGH release doesn't produce any more HGH, making intermittent fasting, not continued fasting, the most effective way to benefit from the release of HGH [Figure 11].

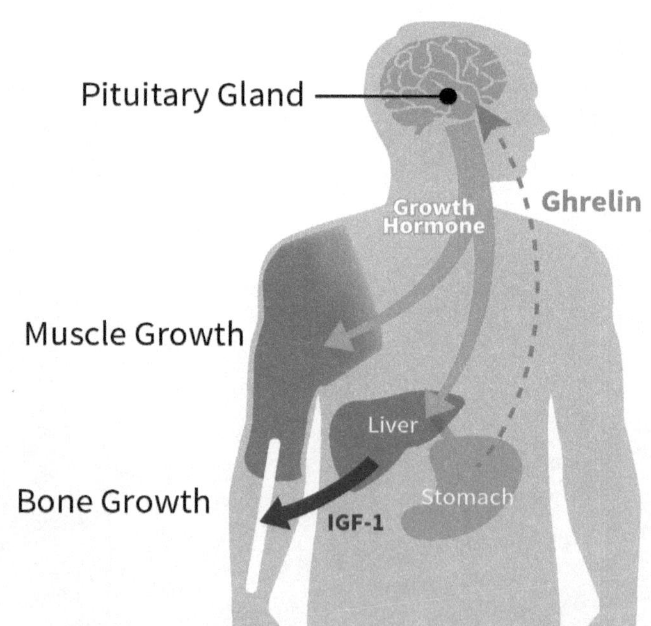

Figure 11 Ghrelin – The Player in Intermittent Fasting

In addition to converting ½ pound of white fat into usable sugar, Human Growth Hormone:

✓ **Activates Thyroid Hormone T4>T3**

✓ **Increases muscle mass (strength)**

✓ **Strengthens bones; preventing and treating osteoporosis and osteopenia**

✓ **Increases tissue production, such as hair, skin and bone**

✓ **Stimulates the growth of all internal organs except the brain**

✓ **Promotes the burning of stored fat and slows sugar storage in the liver and other organs**

✓ **Prevents diabetes**

✓ **Stimulates the immune system**

HGH promotes weight loss by turning ½ pound of white fat into glucose to refill the brown fat compartment. This reverses the fat storage process without ketosis. Call it "metabolic liposuction" [Figure 12]. Think of intermittent fasting, not as a weight loss method, but as a Human Growth Hormone releasing technique.

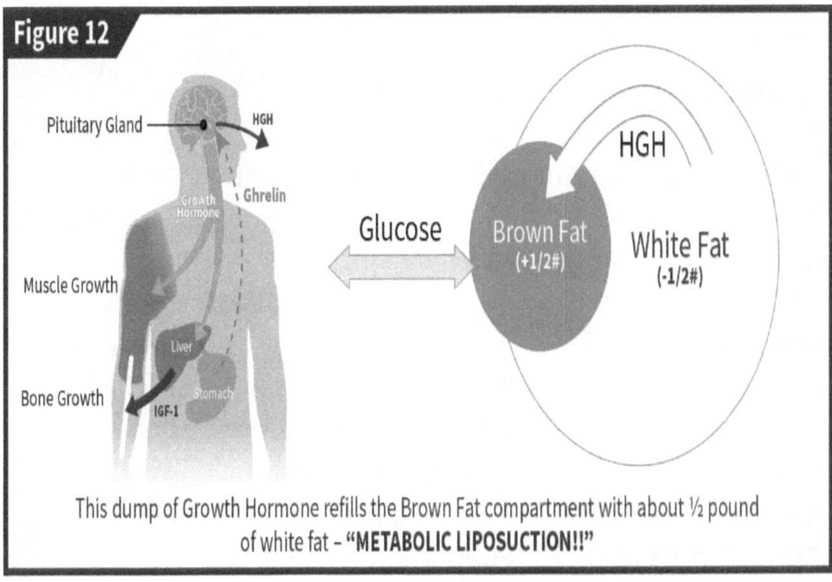

This dump of Growth Hormone refills the Brown Fat compartment with about ½ pound of white fat – **"METABOLIC LIPOSUCTION!!"**

Ghrelin release from the empty stomach, "letting the baby cry" for a while, is a good thing. It has a very positive effect that results in a 20 times normal dump of HGH. Without Ghrelin pulsing the brain cells, HGH is not released. This is the reason for the failure of bariatric surgery and for the temporary effects of gastric balloons. In addition to converting ½ pound of white fat into usable sugar,

Human Growth Hormone:

1. Activates Thyroid Hormone
2. Increases Muscle Mass
3. Strengthens Bones
4. Increases - hair, skin, and bone growth
5. Stimulates growth of internal organs
6. Burns sugars in the liver (fatty liver)
7. Prevents Diabetes
8. Stimulates the immune system

Also, intermittent fasting, besides being the only time we turn white fat directly into glucose, is not associated with the malnutrition that sometimes comes with bariatric surgery and balloon therapy since there is little restriction on the non-fasting days. HGH creams and injections are available but not advised. If HGH is used in excess, it can lead to diabetes. If it is used in smaller amounts, it suppresses your natural release of HGH. Besides, who wants to buy HGH when you can DIY? :)

Section 9
Fasting

Let's say you eat at 8:00 pm and don't snack before bed. By 8am, you are 12 hours into your fast. Ghrelin has been pulsing your brain cells for 12 hours and you probably wake up hungry. On a fasting day, don't eat. Just have some liquid, like coffee or tea. A little cream is OK but don't use non-dairy creamer as it is made of corn syrup solids – i.e. fructose. Drink because you're thirsty, not to stop the hunger feeling. That would be the same as having a balloon stretch the stomach and stops the Ghrelin release. If you must, have a bit of egg or some nuts, but don't eat anything with sugar or starch on a fasting day. This blocks your Leptin and Ghrelin is less restrained making the fasting much, much more difficult. Even eating meals high in starch and sugar the day before a fasting day will make fasting more difficult. Your Ghrelin "baby" will be crying for food by noon. We recommend a sip of water, a little coffee or a bit of egg to pacify the little one. Be reassured, you know that food will be available soon; ask your Ghrelin "baby" to be patient. If your "baby" is in a screaming fit to eat, a little "paci" will get you through the tough spots. As the day goes on, allow the Ghrelin release to do its thing. You will get very hungry on a fasting day, but as you adopt this lifestyle it gets easier to fast. Most of my patients say it begins to feel good, even normal, to be a little hungry. Patients commonly state that they have a renewed clarity of thought. The "sugar fog" lifts. Ghrelin is known to have a strong effect in the hippocampus, which has a role in cognition, adaptation to change and capacity to learn [32]. Ghrelin also has a major role in memory performance.

SECTION 10
THE HUNGER BREAK
"METABOLIC
LIPOSUCTION"

As you practice intermittent fasting, you'll soon realize that when your HGH release occurs, your hunger disappears. Call it the "hunger break", for lack of a better term. You've just changed white fat into glucose to refill the brown fat compartment. "Metabolic Liposuction", a process that is much more natural than surgery, balloons, or counting calories. In addition, you get the many positive effects of HGH. You've forced the fat storage process into reverse, changing ½ pound of that stubborn white fat into glucose in the process! High Five!   You've just completed a 25-mile marathon without taking a single step! Good for you! Good discipline. It's not that exercise isn't good for you - It is!! It's just not an effective tool for weight loss. On non-fasting days, have some breakfast. Keep in mind HFCS will keep you from being satisfied. Cereals and grains will also block Leptin and increase your appetite on the non-fasting days. On the non-fasting days, you are building up human growth hormone (HGH) supply. There is no need to count calories. You are not dieting. Just avoid the foods that make you hungry. If you have a strong desire to eat carbs, do it, but keep in mind they block Leptin and release Ghrelin and that makes you hungrier than you normally would be, you over eat.   EAT NO FRUCTOSE. Then, in one or two days, fast again. Pick out two to three days a week and stick with those. Make it a habit; a part of your lifestyle.

The researchers looking to cure obesity suggest every other day fast (EODF) to cycle brown fat as much as possible. With an odd numbered 7-day work week, I find it hard to make EODF a habit. Besides, I like to relax with family and friends on weekends and food is a big part of socialization. However, if you are OK with EODF, go for it. I fast on Monday and Thursday and avoid sugars and starches on the rest of the days. This is a remnant of the "5-2 fast" that I started with years ago. I was told to lose 45 pounds by my cardiologist. He wanted me to start statins to lower my cholesterol, My A1c was nearly 6 (pre-diabetic). I was eating low fat and exercising every day. The statins made my muscles ache. I heard of the 5-2 fast, got the book and read it. The "5-2" diet allows up to 500 calories a day, but no more, and you do it two days a week. It was a diet - counting calories, watching my weight. It didn't work, Ghrelin is not released long enough, and Leptin remained suppressed. As you make this change in lifestyle, keep in mind: Low carb diet decreases the appetite. Recognize the low-fat foods increase appetite because the fat is replaced with starch "binders" that taste like fat. Eat full fat and get as much HFCS out of the diet as possible. A low-fat diet is associated with five times the risk of the ketodiet. "Pilot studies" are being planned to see if that is really the case. These studies may be available within the next decade. Most of my patients don't have the luxury of waiting a decade to see if they are on the "right" diet.

      We have vast amounts of science to call upon to guide changes in the way we live. The health history of the United States has proven to the world that a low-fat diet, high in fructose is very unhealthy, if not dangerous. This contradicts the advice of some very well-known research organizations and pharmaceutical companies that are "dedicated" to our health.

References

[1] James WP The epidemiology of obesity: the size of the problem. J Intern Med 263: 336–352, 2008.

[2] Mokdad AH, Bowman BA, Ford ES, Vinicor F, Marks JS, Koplan JP. The continuing epidemics of obesity and diabetes in the United States. JAMA 286: 1195–1200, 2001.

[3] Mokdad AH, Ford ES, Bowman BA, Dietz WH, Vinicor F, Bales VS, Marks JS. Prevalence of obesity, diabetes, and obesity-related health risk factors, 2001. JAMA 289: 76–79, 2003.

[4] Mokdad AH, Serdula MK, Dietz WH, Bowman BA, Marks JS, Koplan JP. The continuing epidemic of obesity in the United States. JAMA 284: 1650–1651, 2000.

[5] Mokdad AH, Serdula MK, Dietz WH, Bowman BA, Marks JS, Koplan JP. The spread of the obesity epidemic in the United States, 1991–1998. JAMA 282: 1519–1522, 1999.

[6] Adair LS Child and adolescent obesity: epidemiology and developmental perspectives. Physiol Behav 94: 8–16, 2008.

[7] Bray GA, Nielsen SJ, Popkin BM. Consumption of high-fructose corn syrup in beverages may play a role in the epidemic of obesity. Am J Clin Nutr 79: 537–543, 2004.

[8] Havel PJ Dietary fructose: implications for dysregulation of energy homeostasis and lipid/carbohydrate metabolism. Nutr Rev 63: 133–157, 2005.

[9] Johnson RJ, Segal MS, Sautin Y, Nakagawa T, Feig DI, Kang DH, Gersch MS, Benner S, Sanchez-Lozada LG. Potential role of sugar (fructose) in the epidemic of hypertension, obesity and the metabolic syndrome, diabetes, kidney disease, and cardiovascular disease. Am J Clin Nutr 86: 899–906, 2007.

[10] Basciano H, Federico L, Adeli K. Fructose, insulin resistance, and metabolic dyslipidemia. Nutr Metab (Lond) 2: 5, 2005.

[11] Bray GA, Nielsen SJ, Popkin BM. Consumption of high-fructose corn syrup in beverages may play a role in the epidemic of obesity. Am J Clin Nutr 79: 537–543, 2004.

[12] Johnson RJ, Segal MS, Sautin Y, Nakagawa T, Feig DI, Kang DH, Gersch MS, Benner S, Sanchez-Lozada LG. Potential role of sugar (fructose) in the epidemic of hypertension, obesity and the metabolic syndrome, diabetes, kidney disease, and cardiovascular disease. Am J Clin Nutr 86: 899–906, 2007.

[13] Johnson RJ, Segal MS, Sautin Y, Nakagawa T, Feig DI, Kang DH, Gersch MS, Benner S, Sanchez-Lozada LG. Potential role of sugar (fructose) in the epidemic of hypertension, obesity and the metabolic syndrome, diabetes, kidney disease, and cardiovascular disease. Am J Clin Nutr 86: 899–906, 2007.

[14] Nakagawa T, Hu H, Zharikov S, Tuttle KR, Short RA, Glushakova O, Ouyang X, Feig DI, Block ER, Herrera-Acosta J, Patel JM, Johnson RJ. A causal role for uric acid in fructose-induced metabolic syndrome. Am J Physiol Renal Physiol 290: F625–F631, 2006.

[15] "Database of Select Committee on GRAS Substances (SCOGS) Reviews". Accessdata.fda.gov. 2006-10- 31. Retrieved 2010-11-06.

[16] Rizkalla, S. W. (2010). "Health implications of fructose consumption: A review of recent data". Nutrition & Metabolism. 7: 82. doi:10.1186/1743-7075-7-82. PMC 2991323 . PMID21050460.

[17] M. Ataman Aksoy; John C. Beghin, eds. (2005). "Sugar Policies: An Opportunity for Change". Global Agricultural Trade and Developing Countries. World Bank Publications. p. 329. ISBN Daniels, Lee A. (1984-11-07). "Coke, Pepsi to use more corn syrup". The New York Times. ISSN 0362-4331. Retrieved 2017-01-20.

[18] James Bovard. "Archer Daniels Midland: A Case Study in Corporate Welfare". cato.org. Archived from the original on 2007-07-11. Retrieved 2007-07-12.

[19] Orkaby AR, Cho K, Cormack J, Gagnon DR, Driver JA. Metformin vs sulfonylurea use and risk of dementia in US veterans aged ≥65 years with diabetes [published online September 27, 2017]. Neurology. doi:10.1212/WNL.0000000000004586

[20] Witters LA. The blooming of the French lilac. J Clin Invest. 2001;108:1105–1107.

[21] Hadden DR. Goat's rue - French lilac - Italian fitch - Spanish sainfoin: gallega officinalis and metformin: the Edinburgh connection. J R Coll Physicians Edinb. 2005;35:258–260.

[22] Bailey CJ, Day C. Metformin: its botanical background. Pract Diab Int. 2004;21:115–117. doi: 10.1002/pdi.606.Ben Sahra I, Le Marchand-Brustel Y, Tanti JF, Bost F. Metformin in cancer therapy: a new perspective for an old antidiabetic drug? Mol Cancer Ther. 2010;9:1092–1099. doi: 10.1158/1535- 7163.MCT-09- 1186.

[23] Diamanti-Kandarakis E, Economou F, Palimeri S, Christakou C. Metformin in polycystic ovary syndrome. Ann N Y Acad Sci. pp. 192–198.

[24] Rotella CM, Monami M, Mannucci E. Metformin beyond diabetes: new life for an old drug. Curr Diabetes Rev. 2006;2:307–315. doi: 10.2174/1573399906777950651.

[25] Evans JM, Donnelly LA, Emslie-Smith AM, Alessi DR, Morris AD. Metformin and reduced risk of cancer in diabetic patients. BMJ. 2005;330:1304– 1305. doi: 10.1136/bmj.38415.708634.F7.

[26] Goodwin PJ, Pritchard KI, Ennis M, Clemons M, Graham M, Fantus IG. Insulin-lowering effects of metformin in women with early breast cancer. Clin Breast Cancer. 2008;8:501–505. doi: 10.3816/CBC.2008.n.060.

[27] Algire C, Zakikhani M, Blouin MJ, Shuai JH, Pollak M. Metformin attenuates the stimulatory effect of a high-energy diet on in vivo LLC1 carcinoma growth. Endocr Relat Cancer. 2008;15:833–

[30] "WHO Model List of Essential Medicines (19th List)" (DF). World health Organization. April 2015. Archived (PDF) from the original on 13 December 2016. Retrieved 8 December 2016.

[31] J Clin Invest. Fasting enhances growth hormone secretion and amplifies the complex rhythms of growth hormone secretion in man. K Y Ho, J D Veldhuis, M L Johnson, R Furlanetto, W S Evans, K G Alberti, and M O Thorner, 1988 Apr; 81(4): 968–975.

[32] Heppner KM, Tong J (July 2014). "Mechanisms in endocrinology: regulation of glucose metabolism by the Ghrelin system: multiple players and multiple actions". European Journal of Endocrinology. 171 (1): R21–32. doi:10.1530/EJE-14-0183. PMID 24714083.

[33] Understanding the benefit of metformin use in cancer treatment Ryan JO Dowling,1 Pamela J Goodwin,2 and Vuk Stambolic [34] Diano S, Farr SA, Benoit SC, McNay EC, da Silva I, Horvath B, Gaskin FS, Nonaka N, Jaeger LB, Banks WA, Morley JE, Pinto S, Sherwin RS, Xu L, Yamada KA, Sleeman MW, Tschöp MH, Horvath TL (March 2006). "Ghrelin controls hippocampal spine synapse density and memory performance". Nature Neuroscience. 9 (3): 381–88.

Samuel Tyuluman

36